Sallie Rose MA. L.C.H. is a Homeopath, Life-coach, Writer & Mindfulness Teacher and lives between Hertfordshire and a remote island in Greece. She has attended numerous silent retreats and is committed to help people find quiet spaces in the midst of their busy lives.

Step 1

Mental acceptance

The first step is to really accept that you are in self isolation. This is not the time to reach out to others or engage in your normal activities that have previously provided a structure and meaning to your life. It is a time to withdraw from outward activity and to turn towards yourself.

Whether you do this with a lot of resistance or accept it readily, is up to you. For those of you who always feel the need to be constantly busy this can be extremely challenging. As you embark on this journey, I would ask you to be very gentle and patient with yourself as you enter this unchartered territory.

For others you may already lead quite a solitary life already and this may be your opportunity to approach it in a more engaged and mindful way and even welcome it.

Whatever your circumstances are, instead of seeing it as a time of lack or loss, treat it as a period to:

- Slow down

- Recharge

- Renew

- Nourish

- Connect to yourself and your own natural rhythms

Some of you may have a great deal of self- judgement about spending such an inordinate time concentrating on your own process and experience. Instead, you might want to remind yourself that this experience is not your choice but also that some quiet self-contemplation may be useful and ultimately enhance your relationship both with yourself and others going forward.

Furthermore, although this particular time is somewhat forced upon us, you will find as you go through your life, there might be times when physical illness causes you to take a pause or you decide to take some space for yourself whether this is at home or elsewhere.

The structure that is presented in this book is transferrable can be adapted to many different circumstances and locations. Feel free to adapt it to your own specific needs in that moment of time. For some of you, you may be sharing your living situation with partners or children. If so, you might want to take some of the suggestions from this book and adapt it where you can.

The primary focus of this book is on self-isolation.

Step 2

Establishing self-isolation

The first step is establishing a structure, a container, for this time period of self-isolation. This is symbolic of a moment in time that has a beginning and an end but is outside the normal activities and social interactions in your life. In the following chapters we are going to look at various parts of your container for this time period and help you plan and set up a structure that works for you.

I do encourage you to so all the exercises in this book in longhand as research shows that this helps you really connect to yourself and your specific needs rather than using a screen. I recommend an A5 notebook. However, if this fills you with horror do turn to your computer or laptop instead.

However, if you do the latter, I also advise you to make a boundary that, whilst doing the exercises, you will not check social media or your inbox. There will be plenty of time to do that in other periods of the day. As a long-time procrastinator with a heavy workload I find that establishing a reward system is really useful. So, it might be, for example, that after an hour of intense work or processing I may allow myself fifteen minutes on Facebook. This is your time, so you decide.

Action 1

Establishing your container

Take an A5 notebook and write down on the first page when the time will begin and end. Obviously, your time may be extended but for now just write down the concrete time you are aware of at this time. You might want to do this with a pencil in case the time does change.

> **I** (insert your name) **am entering this self-isolation period from** (start date) **until** (end date).

Action 2

Establishing your intention

When you think of the overall period that lies ahead of you, having gone through the gruelling process of acceptance that it's the way it has to be, I would like you to take some time to think about what your intention is for this period of time.

For some of you, it may be some well needed rest, for others it may be an opportunity to catch up on some forgotten chores, whilst others might welcome the time for gentle reflection to work on some issues, like life choices or dealing with some issues that have been causing you stress or heartache.

Some examples of this may be:

My intention for this retreat is to:

- Increase my health and well being

- Slow down

- Resolve some outstanding issues

- Become comfortable with my own company

- Become more mindful

- Become an avid reader

- Take stock of where I am in my life, and where I want to be

Action 3

Setting your intention

Turn to Page 3 of your A5 book.

Write down the following

My overall intention during this period is to . . .

Review your intention and make sure it's something you

are comfortable with. You can always come back and

change it, and you can have more than one intention, but

focussing on a single, simple, clear goal will provide a

great structure for achieving your intentions.

Step 3

Setting up support and contact

For most people, one of the biggest challenges is the prospect of a long period of time without human contact and interaction. For this reason, it is important to set up a support network of friends and family if you can. I am aware that some people are not so fortunate to have this opportunity but even one person is fine. It is also amazing how supportive neighbours can be at times like this.

Action 1

Regular Contacts

- On page 2 of your A5 notebook, make a list of three people who you are going to have regular contact with during this time. For each person, the regularity of this might be different

- Decide on your means of contact i.e.: messenger app, phone, email, skype, face-time

- Set up specific times to speak at mutually convenient times

(If, on the other hand, you are of a more introverted nature and would prefer to be more self-contained that is fine, but please have at least one person you can call on if needs be.)

Reflection

You might want to really think about when the best time would be for this contact. For some people they like to have the early part of the day for their own personal space and would prefer not to be interrupted. For others, they might like to discuss their plan for the day with one of their contacts. Others might want contact as the day draws to the end.

Whatever happens, make sure you have a list easily available of your doctor and local hospital in case of emergency.

Contact List template

Name	Details	Mode of
contact	Best time	

1

2.

3

Doctor:

Hospital:

Local Pharmacy:

Emergency number:

Grocery online delivery details:

Other important numbers:

Step 4

Supplies

Materials (dependent on your specific needs & budget)

- Food provisions especially fresh fruit and vegetables
- A4 lined & A5 lined or dotted notebook, and any other stationery you might need.
- Pens (stickers, labels etc)
- Playlists
- Yoga mat, dumb bells, blocks, straps
- Foam earplugs
- Headphones
- Pile of books you have always wanted to read (or perhaps now is a good time to signup to kindle unlimited)

- Netflix, prime or some other TV channel for distraction

- House cleaning supplies

- Black bags/ large plastic storage boxes

- Healthy food

- Essential oils, Epsom salts, bubble bath

- Incense, candles

- Warm blanket

- Favourite recipe book

- Garden supplies Inc. seeds, plants, trays, peat pots, trowel, potting compost

Action 1

Make your own personal shopping list

Kitchen needs

Take the time to map out what your food needs will be for the next two-three weeks.

Write down every meal you might want in that time and snacks too.

Now go through the ingredients and combine them together to work out how much of each thing you will need.

Be realistic with yourself, you may need to use less than perfect ingredients, such as long-life milk instead of fresh, but know that you will make the best food you can, even if it's not perfect.

When you have your list go through your cupboards and work out what you already have and what you need to stock up on.

Action 2

Sourcing all supplies

If you are able, go out and buy the supplies you do not have available in your house or order online. If for any reason you are unable to do this, call on one of your support contacts to help you.

You may need to swap out ingredients, and use multiple sources to complete your list, but once ordered you will feel confident and secure that you have your food needs covered.

Step 5

Making a to-do list & Goal Setting

Action 1

Write a to-do list

- Take your A5 notebook and your favourite pen

- Open up your book onto a clean fresh page

- Make a to do list of all the things you have been putting off because you are usually too busy

Examples:

- Putting photos in album

- Movies or box sets you have been meaning to see

- Sending emails/letters to loved ones

- Paperwork in pending pile

- Exercise regime you have been meaning to do
  whether it is Yoga, Pilates, pulling weights

- Books half read, or the pile you have been meaning
  to read

- Recipes you have been meaning to cook

- Sorting/de-cluttering: drawers, wardrobes,
  cupboards, the area under the stairs, loft

- Spring- cleaning

- Setting up a meditation practice

- Journaling/writing

- Craft projects

- Planting tomatoes, lettuce and other veggies

Anything you do not know how to do; you can find an online tutorial to help you.

You will create a list here of things you will need to purchase. Go online and start ordering. Some things will arrive sooner than others, so that will dictate the order you do things so, for example, if your wool for your knitting project comes first, best to work on that project first rather than putting off and waiting for your vegetable seeds to arrive.

Action 2

Tracking your own list

On page 2 of your A5 notebook make your own list according to the template below including:

- Title

- What is actually involved

- How much of a priority it is that it is completed by the end of the self-isolation period out of 1- 10 – (10 being the most important)

An example of the layout is below, feel free to adapt it to something that works for you.

Be creative, there are no wrong ways to do this.

To do List template

Name   **Activities involved**   **Priority**

Completion

Setting a goal

Action 1

Deciding on goals

Go through your **to do** list and then make a list of three more general things you want to achieve during this period.

1. . . . .

2. . . . .

3. . . . .

Here are some examples:

- Become more healthy
- Establish a meditation practice
- Learn something new
- Space & clutter clearing
- Process unfinished business
- Deal with paperwork
- Write that novel, memoir, poem

- Set up that website

- Stretching and fitness

- Make some important decisions about your career and love life

- If you are fortunate enough to have access to a garden; establishing a vegetable patch, tidying the garden...

Goal Setting

To action a goal, it is useful to make it specific and break it down into component parts. The more specific it can be, the easier to follow.

Goals are different to your to do list.

The to do list is things you want to do.

Your goals should be wider, and require multiple things to do to achieve them, so that you can see how your individual activities can contribute to something greater.

Rewards

It is essential to give yourself a reward when you have achieved each goal. Obviously in your self-isolation state it is not going to be possible to buy yourself a treat, but maybe factor in something into your day that may be a reward for you.

Examples of this may be:

- A nice cup of tea or coffee drunk mindfully whilst looking out of the window into the garden or view
- A nice bath with essential oil or bubbles or an energising slow shower with your favourite shower gel
- Playing some relaxation music and doing relaxation exercises
- A nice nap
- Watching a movie, a Tv show or reading a book

* Chatting to your favourite person

Action 3

Your own personal rewards

On P.3 of your A5 notebook, make a list of rewards that you might like to use on achievement of a specific goal.

Now, using your list to help you, take each goal and put it on a separate page of your notebook.
Break it down into easily do-able parts and include the to-dos that lead up to it.

An example of this might be:

1. Decluttering

* Supplies needed e.g.: black bags for waste/charity/labels/ storage boxes

- Decide on what areas need decluttering

- Break down of small decluttering tasks

- Assess how much time you want devote to this task

- Reward when done

2. Planting a garden

- Supplies needed

- Specific things you want to do

- How much time you want to devote to the various tasks

- Reward when done

Inner Work

Some actions may require more considered inner work instead. An example of this may be deciding about a career change or processing some grief around a lost loved one. In this case, your action step may look more like this one:

3. Deciding whether to change your career

- Make a pros and cons list of your current job
- Make a list in notebook of all career options
- Spending an allotted amount of time researching on the internet at availability, training courses or any other relevant information
- Update resume
- Complete a career plan
- When you have done all your research you might want to allot a decision- making session. More about this later . . .
- Reward when done

Step 6

Setting up a structure for your day

This is an extremely important step and requires you sitting down with your notebook and a large piece of paper.

Take a few minutes to breathe and centre yourself and think of how you would like to structure your day taking into account the ebbs and flows of your energy. For some people this may feel too controlled and you would prefer more flexibility. In this case, you may prefer to decide in the moment what to do next. I personally find a structure works as a container and as you enter this quiet time, you may decide to change the structure – nothing is set in stone!

Action 1

Breaking up your day

1.Divide each day into sections that work for you.

See the following template and adapt it to make it your

own.

Sample Timetable

8-9 am: Gentle stretching/yoga

        Journaling

9-10 am: Breakfast and ablutions

10-11 am: Checking in with somebody on your list

/reading

11 am-1pm: Sorting out paperwork

1pm: Lunch

2-4 pm: Nap

4-6 pm: Gardening

6pm: Dinner

7-9 pm: Netflix/ Reading

9pm: Preparing for sleep

2. Make a graph of your energy levels and when it is best for you to do something more physical, and when it might be best to rest. An example of this may be to have a siesta after lunch.

3. Fill in the spaces for each day referring to your previous lists and activities. Some of you might only wish to fill in the first day and sit down that night and plan for the next day. There is no set way to do this, you are tuning into your own unique rhythms and intuition.

Remember none of this is set in stone and can be finely tuned during your period of isolation. You might even want to experiment with times of structure, open time periods and assess for yourself what works best for you. For some of you, your attention span is very short and you may wish to allot certain activities within a smaller time space, others may want more time for each activity.

Also, some of you might be filled with a sense of dread about making your time so structured. If this is the case, you may choose to check in with yourself at a certain time during the day and ask yourself what you would prefer to do at a specific time.

Step 7

Self-reflection

In your notebook, make a page for each day with the time slots and activities.

At the bottom make a space for your reflections on that day.

An example of this might be:

- Mood fluctuations

- Focus

- Difficult moments – examining what triggered them

- Anything particular that came up for you

- How you felt after speaking to a particular person

- What you achieved?

- What you would have done differently?

- Any insights?

***

Feel free to add any additional things that you would find useful.

* * *

Healthy Habits

Some people make a record of healthy habits they would like to keep e.g.:

- Drinking lemon water in the morning
- Having a certain amount of food and vegetables
- Meditating each day

It is your retreat and your page, use it as you will.

Step 8

Yoga & Meditation

Simple Yoga Routine

On the following page is a brief list of a sequence of yoga exercises that you might find useful.

There are countless sites and videos online that will demonstrate them in more detail.

These exercises can be done before or after meditation, or later on in the day.

Please be mindful of any particular ailments and injuries and finely tune the exercises for your own particular needs.

Yoga Sequence

1. **Savasana variation** - Lying on back with knees bent, connecting to abdominal breathing through the nose

Stay in each of the following postures for at least 5 breaths as above

2. **Apanasana** - Hugging knees to chest and rocking from side to side

3. **Jathara Paravitti** - Lying down twist

4. **Bidalasana** - Cat/Cow pose

5. **Ardho Mukha Svasana** - Down Dog with knees bent

6. **Uttanasana** – Standing forward fold with legs hip width and knees bent

7. **Tadasana** – Standing mountain pose, grounding through feet

8. **Parsva Urdhva Hastasana** – standing half-moon pose/side bend

9. **Garudasana & Gomukhasana arms -** Roll down through forward bend, down dog, all fours and onto belly

10. **Salamba Bhujangasana** - Sphynx

11. **Balasana** – Pose of the child

12. Savasana or Savasana variation

Maybe put some music on and let your body sink away for 5/10 mins, or go through a tense and relax from the toes upwards.

Mindfulness Meditation

The best time to meditate is as early as possible in the day before the day becomes flooded with sensory impressions.

It is important to choose a place in your house or flat where you go to regularly.

Even if you live in one room you can make a sacred space there with a chair or cushion, some flowers, a picture of a loved one or pet. If you live somewhere quite noisy you may want to use earplugs.

If you wish, you can start with some gentle stretching to help you ground yourself and become more embodied.

Then set an alarm for a specific amount of time. If you are

new to this practice you may want to only do 5-10

minutes. If you are a more experienced meditator you may

want to extend it to 20-40 minutes. If possible, make sure

the alarm has a gentle sound so the transition back at the

end of your sitting is a gentle one.

Then, take your seat on your chair or your cushion and

establish a dignified posture.

It is best to close your eyes if you feel comfortable with

this.

Make contact with the rise and fall of your belly and the

breath comes and goes.

See how long you can stay with it and when your mind

wanders gently but firmly bring it back to the anchor of the

breath. As you continue, thoughts, feelings and body

sensations will come and go, your task is to remain with

the primary object of the breath. I often liken this to seeing oneself as a tree in a storm. The branches are ruffled by the changing weather but the trunk and roots remain firm and steady.

If you find that you have been pulled away by a particular thought or body sensation, it doesn't matter how long you have been pulled away, the practice is to notice that you went away and bring yourself back.

If you wish, you can connect to some of my own guided meditations.

These can be found on:

https://meditationow.co.uk/mp3s/

Please note I also offer Skype sessions in Mindfulness Meditation instruction, if you feel you need some guidance:

https://meditationow.co.uk/private-sessions/

Step 9

Journaling & other writing exercises.

Journaling

Best to be done as early in the day as possible.

There are many ways to journal and an abundance of books on the subject. If you already have your own method, feel free stick to that. Otherwise, you may find this method useful.

Take your favourite pen. It must be one that you feel at ease writing with so as not to interrupt your flow.

Take an A4 lined notebook and begin writing longhand whatever comes into your mind, without censoring for three pages, and without stopping. Put on paper whatever comes to mind, even if it is an angry outburst or a sudden wave of grief or a memory or a dream. There are no rules other than to keep the pen on the paper and keep writing.

At the end of the session, you may look through it and migrate a particular word or image to use in some other piece of work, or you may choose not to read it at all. It is merely a tool to focus your imagination and get more in touch with yourself.

Decision making

This needs to be done in the second half of your retreat period, and after you have done all your research re your various options.

Action

- Take a new page in your notebook

- Make the title of your decision

- Make a list of options

- For each option make a list of pros and cons.

- Reduce your list to your remaining options

- Light a candle/incense or find another way to be calm

- Go to your special meditation space

Take each option and close your eyes and sit with it. Visualise living it in its entirety and what it would look like, and then feel how you are feeling about it, using 1-10 as the range – one feeling the worst and ten feeling the best.

Continue with each option until you are clear which one is the best for you. There is no wrong answer.

Grieving/letting go of a situation or person

This is probably best done in the second half of the isolation period when you have developed a more balanced and grounded relationship with yourself.

- Set up a time period in your day where you can really connect to yourself.

- Maybe have one of your support system on call just in case you need some extra support

- Make your space warm and comfortable, wrap yourself in a blanket if needed

- Light some candles, burn some oils or incense. Play some music that maybe reminds you of this person

- Wrap yourself up and turn on the music. Take your A4 notebook and begin writing whatever comes up, connected to this person. If a particular emotion comes up try and be with yourself with compassion as if you are your own most beloved child. Tears may come, anger may arise, let each emotion arise and try and stay with it with utter acceptance and compassion

- If it feels too much stop, and maybe slowly walk around the room or do some gentle exercise

- When you feel complete record in your notebook your experience, noting if something has shifted as a result of the exercise

Step 10

Planting a Garden

Apart from the budget needed to buy the seeds or
vegetable plants, there is no reason that you cannot grow
some edible plants regardless of your space.
It is possible to stack plants on a window-sill, up the
vertical sides of a balcony, or if you are lucky enough to
have a garden, you can plant your own vegetable patch.

Window sill

- Buy seed trays or small pots. There are peat pots
  available which can easily be transported into the
  ground when big enough if you have space

- Add some peat or potting compost almost to the top
  and spray with water Gently add the seeds allowing
  for space between them if you can. Cover with a in
  layer of potting compost and spray every day

- These can be transported into your garden or pots, if you have a patio or balcony or into larger pots on your window sill

Garden

- Find a spare patch of ground, or if you want to separate your patch order three railway sleepers and cut the third one in half

- Make a rectangle with the sleepers and fill it with organic compost if possible. This can be ordered online or bought from a garden centre or if you are lucky enough to have a farm nearby or a riding stable. They are usually more than happy to let you collect a few sacks

- Plant your vegetables (either bought, ready grown, or grown from seed) with enough space for each to grow. You might wish to buy a book on companion planting as each family of plants aids the other's growth and helps combat pests

Finally, the things that plants need most to help

them grow and thrive is light, water and above all

TLC (Tender Loving Care)

Step 11

Wellness & nutrition

There is much that can be said about this subject but certainly the most important is to eat healthily at this time. As you will see if you review the literature in this area there is no diet that fits all. For some people a vegan or vegetarian diet may be best, but for others some lean meat and fish may feel necessary. As with everything else during this time, it is important to check in with yourself and really feel what your body needs.

The more you can eat fresh fruit and vegetables and gentle proteins the better.

The foods to avoid generally are the following:

- Processed carbs

- Foods containing Sugar

- Heavily fried foods

- Very sweet or salty sauces

- Concentrated fruit juices

- Excessive dairy

- Red meat

- Excessive caffeine

- Unless you have weak kidneys try and drink at least two litres of water a day

Mindful eating

So often we are distracted when we eat, often doing a few other things at the same time like looking at our screens or even speaking on the phone. Now is an opportunity to slow everything down. Perhaps pick a favourite spot to eat, looking out the window or allowing a shaft of sunlight to fall on your shoulders. Eat slowly, try not to rush and savour every taste, maybe taking a moment to consider the source where the food originally came from.

Bathing and Showering

If you have a bath make sure you use some relaxing and uplifting essential oils, Magnesium flakes or Epsom salts. If you have a shower make sure you take time to feel the burst of water on every part of your body. Make it a ritual

and enjoy every moment.

Preparing for sleep

- Prepare for bed slowly

- Burn some essential oils like Vetivert, Lavender,

  Chamomile & Francincense

- Make sure you dim the lights, and make sure that

  you have stopped any interaction with screens at

  least half an hour before you prepare to sleep

- Make sure the room is well-aired and not too hot.

  Don't listen to the news or have any difficult

  conversations before retiring

- Remind yourself of how important sleep is for renewing and refreshing yourself

- If there is something weighing on your mind you may want to put it on paper as just externalising it can help you detach from it and let it go

- You might choose this time to review your day in the notebook – acknowledging the more challenging times, and also where you experienced some peace and calm

- Now would be the time to maybe set the timetable for the following day if that would be helpful

Step 12

Bringing it all together and re-entering the world

On the last day of your self-isolation retreat, allow yourself time to go through your daily activities and comments and review your time.

Make a list of:

- Things that had been challenging

- Things you have learnt

- Any changes, transformations or realisations

Make an affirmation going forward, something that you want to carry back into your life.

Let your transition back into the world be a gentle one. Take it a step at a time, an encounter at a time, a conversation at a time. If you notice that you are being pulled out of yourself or becoming overwhelmed, plan time in the day where you can retreat, even if it is just for a few minutes. And remember there is always that place to return to even for five minutes, five hours or five days.

Make the best of being allowed to be in the wider world again, connect with friends, take time in nature, appreciate the abundance of sensory input that is around you everywhere.

Be well!

Acknowledgements

- Adoni Patrikios my son, who gave me this idea and used his wonderful IT skills to make it happen.

- Sunnah Rose my daughter, who is a wonderful Yoga teacher and wrote the Yoga Sequence

- Claire Gibson, Peter brown & Jonny Finchum who have given me feedback on this book, many thanks to you.

- Twinkle, my ever-patient cat who has been pretty much ignored while I wrote this.